Positive Thinking
&
Happiness

MANJEET KAUR, PhD

POSITIVE THINKING

DEDICATION

I dedicate this book to the Almighty GOD and my
loving family.

CONTENTS

ACKNOWLEDGMENTS

I thank my husband, Harry, and my two lovely daughters, Ajooni and Alicia, for their unconditional love and support.

Preface

Each one of us would like to be happy and lead a stress free life. It is in our hands to be able to reduce and deal with the anxieties in our lives. This requires relaxing the mind for a few minutes every day, looking at the positive in every situation, and making a choice to be happy when faced with challenging situations. We want to emerge as winners when faced with stress! By learning to accept all situations and looking at the positive that comes out of each situation, we can live a more peaceful life. In order to keep our emotions healthy, we should appreciate the simple moments of life and enjoy all the small pleasures that life has to offer.

In today's fast paced world, we are running around trying to meet the demands of life and squeeze in as much as we can into our daily routines. While fulfilling the demands of our daily lives, we should be prepared to cope with and tackle the hassles that come with our day-to-day life. Being mentally, physically and spiritually strong will provide a cushion for us to be able to bounce back from life's pressures and fight the stresses of life.

Life nowadays is dependent a lot on technology. The tasks that came to us naturally a few decades ago, like playing outdoors, going for walks with friends and family, sharing jokes, and laughing together, are now replaced by internet, cars, television, and cell phones. Life is moving too fast, we need to slow down to enjoy the amazing and wonderful natural environment around us. In addition to regular exercising and maintaining a good diet, it is very important to look at the positive in all situations and be happy in order to lead a worthwhile life.

In this book, I am sharing the techniques that have helped me become and remain a happy person in face of multiple stresses in my life. Spending just 20 to 30 minutes regularly on the techniques mentioned in this book has helped me in leading a more happy and meaningful life. I have been practicing positive thinking and happiness techniques regularly by using many different approaches, such as: breathing exercises, traditional yoga, meditation, positive yoga, and happy visualization. Practicing these, I have been blessed with a new me who is ready and strong to tackle problems and challenges.

Like most of us, I too have had a lot of stress in my life. However, I am grateful for all the stress in my life because it has taught me to stay strong and appreciate what I have. In order to maintain a balance in life, for all that we receive, we need to give back a little to the universe. I have learned to accept and deal with the stressful situations by working on what is in my control, and not worrying about what I cannot control. If it weren't for the stresses in my life, I would not be the happy, loving and grateful person I am today.

The ups and downs of life have made me a fighter. I have become an accepting person who is extremely optimistic. I am very happy with these changes since they have made me more relaxed, optimistic, confident, and strengthened my faith in the power of positive thinking for the attainment of happiness.

I hope you enjoy reading this book and wish you will be able to apply these techniques to achieve overall wellness. Happy reading! ☺

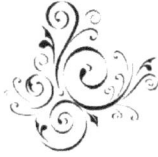

Chapter 1

POSITIVE THINKING

What we think, we become.
All that we are arises with our thoughts.
With our thoughts, we make the world.
                                        - The Buddha

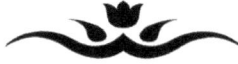

When I concentrate on the positive in everything, I see it in a positive light

This leads the way to hope and makes everything seem possible and bright

In this brightness, I glow with positive energy, and seek contentment

It is this light that helps me attain fulfillment and paves the way to enlightenment

My brain is the organ that perceives the outside world based on my senses

It sends messages to the rest of the body, which prepares my body for defenses

When I train the brain to think above, far and beyond, then

I, only I, will enjoy the pleasures of the mind, body and spirit, it strengthens

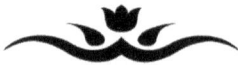

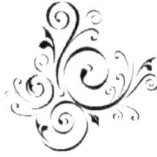

I think, act and behave based on MY perceptions

LET'S CONTROL OUR THOUGHTS BEFORE THEY CONTROL OUR LIVES

In order to face the stresses of life and emerge a winner in challenging situations, it becomes important for us to feed our minds with loving positive thoughts, and nourish the body and soul with meditation. Wisdom lies in opening the heart and mind and embracing all that comes with life. But where does this wisdom come from? Our brains! How do we feed that wisdom into our brains? For me, the answer has been by practicing positive thinking. Having positive thoughts and being optimistic leads to relaxation and happiness in life.

The old proverb - *Practice makes perfect* - applies very aptly to our health and wellness, which is governed by our brains. If we learn to control our minds, we can guide our brains to perceive positive in everything, including the positive and negative situations. Negative emotions create havoc in our body. In order to be disease-free, we need to send positive messages to our bodies so that our brain-body connection can create a path of relaxation and let the flow of energy within our bodies run smoothly without any bumps. To move forward, we need to concentrate on positive thoughts and emotions, and break away from the thoughts that tax our nervous system.

3

To think positive, the *mind* has to be under an individual's control, rather than controlling the individual. We control our minds. In any kind of situation, our thoughts are flooded with positive and negative emotions. Concentrating on the positive emotions leads to more self-control. When we are more in control of our emotions we are more stable emotionally, our senses are more alert, and we can look at things more positively. The mind can be trained through meditation to have faith in the positive energy and spiritual power within each one of us; it can be trained to look at the positive side of situations and individuals alike. What comes out of this training is a HAPPY and RELAXED person. When we are in a positive and happy state of mind, the positive energy itself guides all our life decisions and paves the way to success. The power lies within us. We use only one percent of the powerful energy we are bestowed with, the rest remains unused. The more we use this positive energy, the more power we get to control our thoughts and guide them towards positive outcomes. If we connect to positive energy by practicing relaxation techniques and meditation, we can attract good fortune.

Life is a journey filled with joys and sorrows. Throughout life we come across different and difficult situations which we cannot simply ignore. We have to look at what makes us happy and adopt ways of life that will lead to a satisfying and fulfilling journey. Would one lay more emphasis on that which leads to negative emotions and makes life miserable, or would one search for how to deal with the situation in a way that will solve our problems and help us avoid these in the future? Once we tackle a stressful situation, it will no more be a challenge for us.

The secret lies in accepting the challenging situation and gearing our thoughts towards positivism so that we are more in control of ourselves. Only then we can enhance problem solving skills to make rewarding decisions.

Advantages of Thinking Positive

1. Individuals who think positive are able to deal better with stress since they approach every situation with an optimistic attitude.

2. By thinking positive, we gain insight into optimal living, which optimizes our ability to deal with challenging situations and enhance positivism in all spheres of life.

3. Positive thoughts help us understand our emotions and psychological concepts at a deeper level.

4. Increase in positive emotions leads to well-being and helps us to live life to the fullest by always being happy.

5. Positive thinking leads to mental, physical, spiritual, and financial wellness and helps in acquiring a better understanding of individual and cultural differences.

We keep learning throughout our life; with learning we acquire new traits and characteristics that further nourish our consciousness and soul. Be it joy or sorrow, every human being experiences the emotions involved. When challenging life situations arise, we have to make choices to deal with those situations. If we give in, we have already failed the test. If we accept the challenging situation, look at the positive and move forward to tackle it, we have half won the battle.

<u>Acceptance</u>

Accepting situations and people is the first step towards problem solving. If we learn to accept both the joys, and sorrows of life, we will be in a better position to maintain a balance in our lives. When distressed, we should gather our thoughts and devise strategies which will lead to positive outcomes.

Why fret when it will negatively affect our health and only lead to regret?

It helps to surrender to life itself by accepting and being compassionate in healing the wounds it gives us. If we treat the wounds with love, the healing will be faster.

We build our own personalities based on past experiences. What and how we think, feel and act become lasting traits and build our unique personalities. If our love is stronger than our negative feelings, we will develop a loving personality.

Being happy doesn't mean that everything is perfect. It means that you have decided to look beyond the imperfections.

- Gerard Way

HELPFUL TIPS

Food for Thought

Think about two challenging situations in your life – one in which you achieved success, and another in which you had to struggle a lot, but were still unsuccessful?

Challenging situation with a successful outcome	Your reaction	Outcome
Challenging situation with an unsuccessful outcome	Your reaction	Outcome

The outcome of each situation might throw some light on how you responded in each case. Do you think responding differently might have helped? For example, if you would have been more relaxed, would you have had a different outcome?

<u>Forgiveness</u>

Forgiving others and ourselves is the next step to take after acceptance. Almost all our emotional experiences involve others. Many times, knowingly or unknowingly, we hurt our loved ones and also get hurt ourselves by others. In instances like this, learning to forgive heals the emotional wounds faster. Forgiveness takes us closer to achieving fulfillment and connecting further to the positive flow of energy inside us.

To err is human; to forgive, divine
- Alexander Pope

When we ourselves make mistakes, we should not hold grudges against others. I believe, by forgiving others, we forgive ourselves.

<u>Optimism</u>

The best way to keep ourselves going and deal with the stresses before they overcome us, is to look at the positive in every situation. See the good in every situation and be hopeful of the best results. Sometimes, it becomes very difficult to look at something positive in a very stressful situation. In cases like that, we need to remember that dwelling on the negatives and worrying too much about the outcomes will only weaken us and lead to illness and disease. If we think and look for the positive in this kind of stressful situation, we are sending a positive message throughout our body as well.

For myself I am an optimist - it does not seem to be much use being anything else.
- Sir Winston Churchill

<u>Train the Brain</u>

One of the greatest treasures humans have is the power of thinking. We have no control over what life throws at us, but we do have control over how we receive and respond to it. What guides us in that? Our BRAIN! The brain has to be trained to form positive habits by regular practice. To form a new habit, we need to break the old ones. In order to break the old habits, we have to practice the new habit for at least a month or so, to bring about a permanent change in our behavior and make the new habits a part of our lifestyle.

We can shape our lives to a great extent if we train our brains to practice positive thinking techniques regularly. Practice mindfulness, meditation and relaxation; the more we practice, the more relaxed and accepting we will become. It should become a way of life. The practice should be regular; if we stop, our mind might start wandering again. Just as we eat, drink and sleep regularly, we need to meditate as well so that we can control our minds and relax our brains, which in turn will relax our bodies and pave the way to mental, physical, and spiritual well-being.

Sometimes, even with regular practice, our minds might wander. Being human, we go through emotions all the time. The success of meditation lies in not becoming desperate and vulnerable, but instead continuously practicing relaxation techniques to calm and control the negative emotions, and enhance positive emotions. When faced with challenges, we need to accept them, control our emotions and work towards achieving positive outcomes.

Creativity

Being creative is the ability to be innovative by conceiving an idea from our imagination. Humans are gifted with the power of thinking. By using the ability to invent ideas with our fertile brains, we can use our imagination and knowledge to come up with unique concepts. For example, if you like to cook, create innovative delicacies by trying new cooking techniques.

Making Dreams and Thoughts Come True

We all dream about achieving success in different spheres of life, but how many of us actually put these dreams and thoughts into action? Success comes to those who believe in fulfilling their dreams and working towards achieving their goals. Achieving fulfillment of dreams is easier than we think. In my experience, it is a simple process:

1. The first step is *action.* First and foremost, in order to tread the path of dream fulfillment, put thoughts into action. Get out of bed every morning with the thought: In order to achieve my goals, I need to first wake up and start working towards putting my dreams into action.

2. The second step is *patience* and *persistence;* keep working diligently till success is achieved, and even after you have reached your goals.

HELPFUL TIPS

Dream Fulfillment

Now is the time to practice fulfillment of your dreams. Think of something you have been wanting to do but have been procrastinating and answer the questions below:

What is my dream?

How do I feel when I think about or dream this dream?

Do I want to make this dream a reality?

What steps will I take to achieve fulfillment of my dream?

　　1.

　　2.

　　3.

How do I feel?　　READY TO ACHIEVE SUCCESS ☺

Easy Steps
DREAM → Put dreams into action → Work diligently → Be patient → Be persistent → **DREAM FULFILLMENT**

Motivation and Leadership

Leadership is a quality and process where an individual comes up with an idea, leads the way to action, convincing other people to follow. The leader, the person who starts the process takes the lead and influences others to follow, working together towards the attainment of a common goal or objective.

Most of us have come across situations in life where while in a group, someone poses a question to the group. Initially, people in the group might be reluctant to answer, but as soon as one person answers, others follow. The leader is this person who put his thinking into action and led the way to the discussion. We all have ideas, however, the leader is the person who puts that idea into action and leads the path, making way for others to tread.

Self Esteem

Abraham Maslow, a famous psychologist, came up with a pyramid where he placed needs according to hierarchy: physiological, safety and security, love and belongingness, self esteem and self actualization (Myers).[1] The fourth need in this pyramid, self esteem is the feeling of regard, approval, and respect for the self which may depend a lot on an individual's environment. When we are surrounded by people who love and admire us, a feeling of love and belongingness is generated, which further raises our morale. When our self-esteem is high, awareness of self brings joy and freedom into our lives. Our focus and concentration increases and we become more involved in what we do, thus achieving success in academic, home, social and occupational fields.

Love, Forgiveness and Generosity

Giving unconditional love, forgiving others and being generous with our love makes other individuals feel more comfortable when dealing with us. If we send out positive vibrations, the same will come back to us. Many times our responses to challenging situations are anger and resentment, which only makes things worse for us. Anger and resentment are not the solution, but one thing is certain, anger affects our bodies in a negative way. Our heart rate and blood pressure go up disrupting the normal flow of blood in our bodies. To keep our body systems running smoothly, it becomes essential for us to feed and train our brains with thoughts that will generate positivism in and around us.

Giving and receiving love, both is a pleasure;
let's share it like the selfless love we receive from our mothers

Our Actions and Behavior Affect Others

We need to treat others the way we want to be treated ourselves. If we are in a challenging relationship situation, acting the way we want others to act, can produce desirable results. For example, if we want others to accept us with our faults, we first need to accept others and give them unconditional love. Controlling our emotions, which guide our behavior, is the first step towards acceptance. By learning relaxation techniques, we train our brain to relax and control our behavior in challenging situations. Accepting what comes our way and learning to deal with it provides support for positive thoughts and happy outcomes.

Our Actions and Behaviors Affect Others	

Let us think of a scenario where two people (I am going to call them Bill and Tom) have planned a family dinner-movie night out. Both have a busy day at work and are late getting home from work due to rush hour traffic.

	BILL	TOM
REACTION ON GETTING HOME	Enters the house in anger, throws his briefcase away and yells at the family for not being ready or some other trivial thing.	Enters the house with a smile, apologizes to the family and asks them to give him a few minutes to freshen up.
RESPONSE OF THE FAMILY	Family gets angry and there is argumentation.	Family smiles back and gives a positive response.
CONSEQUENCES	Bill is angry - family is angry	Tom is relaxed - gets positive response from family - family is relaxed.

HELPFUL TIPS

Thinking Positive Exercise

Step 1: Relax the mind and body; bring a smile to the face.

Step 2: Be aware of why and what you are practicing e.g. positive thinking and awareness.

Step 3: Think of the emotional or physical pain you are going through because of some stressful situation.

Step 4: Think of an emotional or physical pain someone you are close to might have been going through for a while.

Step 5: If you feel your pain is stronger than what most humans go through, meditate more often to become strong. If you feel their pain is stronger, be grateful. Either way, concentrate on the positive in the stressful situation.

For example, if one is suffering from a curable disease, think of diseases that do not give other humans the chance to live. Be optimistic by having confidence in yourself and trust in the therapy.

Easy Steps

POSITIVE THINKING HABITS → Acceptance → Forgiveness → Control Emotions → Train the Brain to Relax → **HAPPY HEALTHY LIFE**

<u>Being Grateful</u>

Living life and enjoying every moment to the fullest; relishing the happy moments and being grateful, brings happiness and contentment in our lives. We need to work on making the stressful moments positive by being optimistic. We can perceive distressing moments as giving us strength and making us stronger by looking at the positive in our problem situation and choosing ways to solve the problem. We can also work on eliminating the negativity in these situations by taking them in our stride and ALWAYS concentrating on the positive by developing an optimistic attitude. Being grateful for what we have paves the way to contentment.

To live a life that is fruitful

A good choice is to be grateful

Best to forget experiences that are painful

Enjoy every moment of life and be restful

HELPFUL TIPS

One Day Gratefulness Practice

For one day, consciously pay attention to your assets and be grateful for everything you have. Practice this morning to evening for just a day. Doing this practice makes us realize how many assets we have and how fortunate we are.

Wake up	Be grateful for being able to get up in the morning, running chores and having a job to go to.
Morning Rush	Be grateful for having food on the table, clothes to wear, and a loving family to satisfy our love and belongingness needs.
Work	Be grateful for having a job, a car to drive to work in and being able to earn money to satisfy your needs and fulfill your desires.
Dinner	Be grateful again for having food on the table, home for shelter and a loving family to come back to.
Sleep	Be grateful for the safety and happiness bestowed on you. Relax the mind, smile and be grateful. Look forward to the next day! ***Sweet Dreams!*** ☺

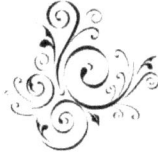

Chapter 2

HAPPINESS

Many persons have a wrong idea of what constitutes true happiness. It is not attained through self-gratification but through fidelity to a worthy purpose.
- Helen Keller

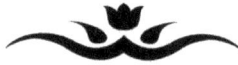

When I am happy, it is obvious from my gait

I do not need anyone, for whom do I wait?

My mind is my best friend, I need to train it to match my thinking chemistry

I will look at the future and remember that past events are history

I will confidently move forward and meet all obstacles with easiness

My best friend, my brain, will guide my happiness.

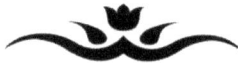

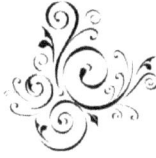

I will practice happiness, the wheel of my life is in MY hands

I CHOOSE TO BE HAPPY

What is happiness? How do I achieve happiness? What is it that makes people happy? What can I do to be happy? Most people are in search of answers to these questions of happiness. But, where do we really find happiness? Happiness comes from our brains, thoughts and actions. It is a state of mind that is associated with contentment, energy, gratitude, joy, love, optimism, positivism, resilience, strength, and well-being.

Happiness is a process, which is attainable by controlling the way we think. Our senses sense stimuli in the environment and send neural messages to our brains. Our brains perceive these messages and send these messages throughout our bodies making us act and behave accordingly. If our brain perceives stimuli as stressful, it will send negative messages to the body; the body in turn will react with increased heart rate, blood pressure and respiration rate paving the way for disease and illness. This is not good for our health.

Looking at the brighter side, if the brain perceives stimuli as challenging, it prepares our body for action. We need to learn to control our thoughts and train our brains

21

to look at the positive in all situations, so that we can make *positive outlook* a habit in life and make lifestyle-thinking changes. Happiness lies in making the right decisions to solve problems.

The universe is set in such a way that there is a balance in everything: up-down, day-night, summer-winter. Our lives run in the same way: awake-asleep, happy-sad, sorrow-joy. As we go through our daily lives, we are faced with so many hassles, right from getting up in the morning - pressing the snooze button, running through morning chores, traffic jams, getting to work, dealing with co-workers and friends, driving back home, taking care of children/parents, preparing dinner and other individualized tasks - till we go to bed at night.

How can we calmly face these challenges in life, one may ask? The answer for me lies in Acceptance and Positive Thinking (APT!) Accepting what comes our way in life and looking for the positive in stressful situations is what will carve the way to happiness. When faced with difficult situations in life, we can attack or cope with the situations in two ways – either give up or face the situation. This is what Walter Cannon called the *fight or flight* response, situations that prepare people to fight or run away from threats (Myers).[1]

If we fight a situation, we do have a chance to win, but if we run away from it, we have already accepted defeat. For example, if an individual loses his/her job and blames the economy, boss or self for the loss, his/her negative thinking will lead to health problems and weaken the ability to look for new jobs. Not only has that person slowed the job search but has also taken the path of negative thinking, which is only going to affect that person solely. On the other hand, if the same individual takes control of the situation and accepts the fact that one needs to move forward, then he/she has half-won over the situation. Rather than getting depressed over the job loss, you look at your skills and take action; you move forward.

I have worked with a diverse population of job seekers helping them to get back into the work force. I learned a lot about happiness in dealing with them. Some individuals actually saw the job loss as an opportunity to look for a new job. They would relate to me how they had stuck to their jobs in spite of long working hours, traveling distances, or dealing with difficult bosses and co-workers. These individuals had accepted the job loss situation, looked at the positive that came out of it, and moved forward with determination. These were the individuals who joined the workforce faster because of their positive attitude. They made the choice to be and remain happy!

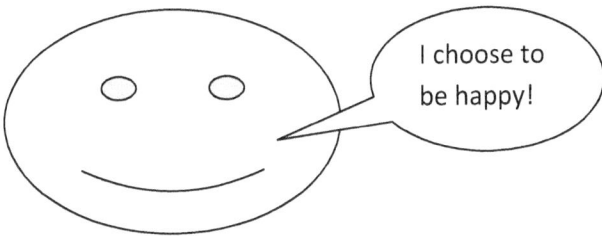

Our perceptions are based on past experiences; our choices are made based on these experiences. If I want to be happy, I have to make the choice to lead a happy life by looking at the positive in each situation and learning from my mistakes.

Even in situations where we see no hope, we sometimes look at that one ray of light which will lead the way to achievement of our goals. If we are searching something in the dark night, come dawn, the first ray of light increases our hope of recovery. Life is such; that one ray of hope will tread the path to reach the goals. It is not easy though. Just like we earn respect, we have to put in a lot of hard work to achieve happiness. The sorrows, failures, lean phases in our lives will always be there and will pull us down. It is we, who make the decision to rise above these situations by controlling our thinking and choosing the happy way to life.

A theoretical model proposed that attainment of happiness is linked to the self...when perception of the self is flexible, happiness seems to be more authentic and durable (Dambrun & Ricard).[2]

Happiness Across Nations

Brazil is a nation that believes in celebrating. Lawmakers in Brazil are coming up with a bill on happiness; a law that protects the pursuit of happiness... The bill before Brazil's Congress would insert the phrase "pursuit of happiness" into Article 6 of the constitution, which states that education, health, food, work, housing, leisure and security - among other issues - are the social rights of all citizens.[3]

I believe that in order to develop adults with a positive outlook on life, they need to be trained in elementary school. It would help to a great extent to include courses on positive thinking, happiness attainment and stress management in the school and college curriculum so that kids learn from an early age.

Spheres of Happiness

Happiness revolves mostly around these factors:

Biological: Good physical health and optimal wellness

Psychological: Relaxed, serene and calm mind

Social: Enduring, positive and happy relationships

Financial: Enough money to enjoy life and pay the bills

Emotional: Being in control of one's emotions when faced with challenging situations.

Spiritual: Relaxation of the brain to get a feeling of being connected to positive energy

Is It Income or Social Support That Makes Us Happy?

Happiness is a search. It is a way of life we choose for our personal satisfaction. Happiness is very subjective and depends a lot on what kind of circumstances we are in.

Can **money** *buy happiness?* Money cannot buy happiness, but money does make us happy when we have enough to use it the way we want to. Think about it, if we have sufficient money to meet all our basic needs, and a little extra to spend it the way we want to, doesn't that make us happy? The answer is subjective.

Authors analyzing American and Japanese participants observed that whereas Americans associate positive hedonic experience of happiness with personal achievement, Japanese associated it with social harmony (Uchida & Kitayama).[4]

A study examining the role of income and social support in predicting happiness and the changes in happiness of married adults over a 10-year period found that income had a small but positive impact on happiness; family social support showed a positive association with concurrent happiness, even after income was controlled (North, Holahan, Moos & Cronkite).[5] Family social support was found to be more strongly associated with happiness when family income was low, than when income was high. Furthermore, change in family social support was positively related to happiness whereas change in family income was unrelated to happiness.

Do Friends and Family Enhance Happiness?

In order to feel and remain happy, we need to be with people who make us feel good about ourselves. All humans are nice and mean good to others, but still many times, even the best of people find it difficult to maintain a relationship. Spending good times with friends makes us feel happy and fulfills our needs for love and belongingness. In that sense, friends do enhance our happiness.

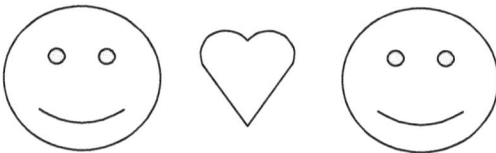

It is said, blood is thicker than water. While family is bestowed on us, we do have control over the friends we make. Many times we feel that friends are everything in the world because we choose them, but time and again, we experience in life how family stands by us when we are in dire need of support. Most of us might have gone through situations where we wanted to help others in need, but just couldn't because of prevailing circumstances. The bonds we make while growing up with our families - going through childhood together, sharing wonderful experiences with our uncles, aunts and cousins - can never be broken. Sometimes, as we grow up, there are personality clashes and stressful situations arise. Nevertheless, we can depend on family to be there for us when we need them. Think positive and positive relationships will build up.

A research study found that two separate types of prosperity – economic and social psychological – best predict different types of well being (Diener & Arora).[6]

Resilience

As we go through life, we experience different kind of emotions based on life situations. We deal with some of these in a very effective manner and move on with life. Some situations are very challenging, however, we still cope with them even though we have to go through many hardships. There are times when things keep happening and we become vulnerable under stress. We might reach a phase in life where we feel pressured from all sides; we get a feeling that life is at a standstill. It is very easy to break down under this pressure, but we need to stay strong and face these challenges. Resilient individuals accept these challenges and rebound to their normal strong self in the face of adversity. If we give in to challenge, we have lost it all, but if we put in the effort and look at how to face these challenges, we have already taken the first step towards success. One big quality of people who reach their goals is that they keep going and do not give up. Hang in there ☺

Research suggests that it is in-the-moment positive emotions, and not more general positive evaluations of one's life, that form the link between happiness and desirable life outcomes. It is further suggested that happy people become more satisfied not simply because they feel better but because they build resources for living well (Cohn, Fredrickson, Brown, Mikels & Conway).[7]

Feel Happy for Others

Each and every individual has the right to be happy; good things happen to all of us. So why do we bask in our own happiness and feel threatened by the happiness of others? Feeling happy for others is an important step towards gaining happiness and peace of our own mind. Feeling delighted by other peoples' happiness and good fortune actually leads to our own serenity and calmness of mind. When we feel happy, the good hormones released in our bodies have a positive effect on our health, which means that if we are constantly happy, we will be healthier. If the opposite happens - we are not happy or are envious of other peoples' good fortunes - our brain and body will be in a state of turmoil leading to irregularities in our body functions. Our feelings of envy actually have no effect on other peoples' happiness but these negative feelings definitely affect our health, happiness and well being.

There are millions of people on this earth; if we feel happy for others, we are increasing our own happiness a million-fold.

The best way to cheer yourself is to try to cheer somebody else up

- Mark Twain

Spending on Others

Spending money on others and living with the joy of being able to help others is more rewarding than spending money just on ourselves.

Recent evidence indicates that spending money with the intention of acquiring life experiences makes people happier than spending money with the intention of acquiring material possessions (Caprariello & Reis).[8]

Findings have suggested that the rewards experienced by helping others may be deeply engrained in human nature, emerging in diverse cultural and economic contexts. Survey data has shown that using financial resources to help others is associated with greater happiness around the world (Aknin, Barrington-Leigh, Dunn, Helliwell & Burns et al.)[9]

Memory

The joyous moments we spend in the company of others and the memories we make stay with us for a lifetime.

Research data has suggested that as related to happiness, relatively unhappy people show somewhat conflicting memorial tendencies whereas very happy people show less conflicting tendencies (Liberman, Boehm, Lyubomirsky & Ross).[10]

Laughter and Humor

Laughter has a lot of healing effects. Statements related to laughter include: laughter is the best medicine, laughter is a natural pain killer, laughter reduces stress.

Laughing more often not only enhances mental and physical health but also helps reduce the fine lines and wrinkles that appear with age.

People who make the choice to remain happy and look for positivity in every situation, tend to be successful in many spheres of life – health, home, work, society and emotional relationships. Happy people attract good fortune and maintain relationships at a deeper level as a result of their positive outlook on life. They are more sociable which makes other people comfortable around them.

Our brains send the same message to the body when we smile for real or fake a smile; the biological and psychological effects are the same. So, it is very important to smile, it has many beneficial effects on our biological, psychological and social functions.

Rejoice in Life's Small Pleasures

Celebrate life! Celebration should not mean spending money, effort and time on a particular occasion. Just being happy and feeling delighted is a celebration in itself. Closing our eyes and bowing in gratefulness is celebration.

Doing something for others and rejoicing in their happiness makes our own happiness double-fold. Sharing the joy of others will give us happiness. When we are happy, our brains relax and that leads to relaxation of the body. Ever paid attention to your glowing face when you have had a good time with family or friends? The brain does not have to feed the body with the message as to why you are happy. Whether we are happy for ourselves or for others, our body will be in the same relaxed state of mind.

Happiness comes from being our natural self. Every individual has a unique personality type and we all act, feel and behave according to our perceptions. Since no two individuals have exactly the same personality, why compare? Every human has strengths and weaknesses. Just as others accept us with our shortcomings, we should try our best not to pay attention to their negatives, instead look for positive qualities and traits in others. After all, nobody is perfect.

Living in the Present Moment

Every moment in life that gives us happiness is a moment to celebrate. Every moment that passes is a thing of the past. Being actively involved in what is happening in the present moment and living it to the fullest is what leads to a happy and pleasure filled life.

Living in the present moment, becoming involved, and enjoying simple pleasures of life leads to a happy life. We can derive immense pleasure while performing daily rituals and simple tasks. Let's take an example of going for a morning walk. In addition to reaping the physical benefits of walking, we can mentally and spiritually enjoy the environment around us and become involved in the creations of the Universe. Looking at the sky, trees, landscapes, enjoying the scenic beauty, smiling at strangers going by, getting obstacles (stones, rocks, sticks) out of the way, helping kids or seniors – all these will bring a smile to our face and add to our spiritual and mental health. On a regular basis, if we practice and concentrate on what leads to happiness, we will become happy individuals.

<u>Characteristics of Happy People</u>

Happiness can be achieved by practicing certain mental tasks and rituals and making them a part of our cognitive ability. Based on research and my personal experience, I feel that if we concentrate on the following on a regular basis, we can achieve happiness.

1. Accept challenges
2. Be grateful
3. Be optimistic
4. Celebrate precious moments of life
5. Enjoy life's small pleasures
6. Exercise daily
7. Increase altruistic behavior
8. Laugh more often
9. Spend quality time with family and friends
10. Show commitment
11. Think positive

In concluding this chapter on happiness, I would like to say, happiness comes from within us. The decision is ours, we can choose to be happy in all situations, even ones that bother us. When we are happy within, we can overcome anxiety and depression, deal better with stressful situations and nourish lasting and loving relationships in all spheres of life. Learning and choosing to be happy and relaxed when distressed, also helps us to deal with, and heal to a great extent, stress-related illnesses like allergies, anxiety, asthma, diabetes, digestive problems, high cholesterol, hypertension, insomnia, tiredness and sexual problems.

When faced with problems, our success in dealing with the problems lies in being bold and facing the problems rather than running away from them. Just like when we try to remove an obstacle from a path we are walking on, in the same way we need to take action to deal with obstacles in our life path. For example, if you are walking on a side walk and see a rock that might hurt other walkers, it is best to stop, give it a thought, and remove the obstruction if it is in your, and others, best interest. Once the obstacle is removed, we can walk on the smooth surface. Similarly, once a challenging life situation is dealt with, we can move forward smoothly in life, taking care of problems as they come. Yes, this is life; problems will be there. Hey, like they say, never a dull moment...keep going.

I believe, what works best is to make the choice to be happy by being optimistic and looking at the positive in all situations. Relax by meditating regularly and you will be immensely pleased with the results.

☺

HELPFUL TIPS

Steps to Achieve Happiness

Happiness for me involves the following steps:

Step 1: Perceive the situation in a positive light

Step 2: Be optimistic and assess the situation

Step 3: Search for the positive outcomes in that situation

Step 4: Achieve success by acting on it in a productive manner

Step 5: Learn from it, to prepare for the future.

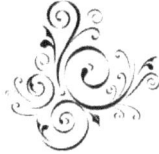

Chapter 3

RELAXATION AND STRESS MANAGEMENT FOR ADULTS

In times of great stress or adversity, it's always best to keep busy, to plow your energy into something positive.

- Lee Iacocca

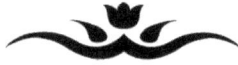

When everything in life goes well, I feel blessed

A small change in life leads to stress

Everything seems to be in a mess

To a child's state, I digress

One thing goes wrong, and I feel bereft;

the wrong notion is that all will be well if I wept

If at that moment, I control my thoughts and progress

to approach the problem with dignity,

I will achieve success!

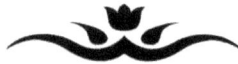

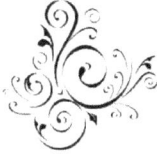

Relaxation, coping MY WAY with daily hassles and life stresses

TRAIN THE BRAIN TO THINK POSIITVE

We all are used to living life according to a certain routine that we have set for ourselves. When changes happen in our life, they require a change to that routine, which often leaves us feeling threatened and challenged. This stress can be related to one's physical self, psychological well-being, social relationships, work challenges, health and wellness, and the environment. To face these challenges we have to put in more effort and energy in order to cope with the new situation; this is what leads to stress. In order to solve problems, we might need to think more, which means using our brain more, or we might have to use extra physical energy as well.

As we go through life experiences, our brains automatically become programmed to the ways we sense and perceive stimuli in our environment. The information our brains receive from the outside world through our senses, is processed by the brain, which then sends messages to the body, making the body behave accordingly. For example, if you take a certain route to work every day, but one day, your mind is preoccupied with something that is bothering you, you still reach your work destination without having paid conscious attention to the roads and traffic signals. Scary, isn't it? This happens because our brains become programmed to follow the familiar roads every day. In the same way, all our behavior is programmed in our brains, the way we behave, is learnt.

Now, there is good stress and there is bad stress. Examples of good stress are getting a promotion, buying a new home, getting married, or going on vacation. All these things make us happy, but we need to make changes to our daily routines to enjoy this good stress. Getting a promotion might mean having to put in more hours at work or moving into a new office. With the extra money one gets from the promotion, one might want to now buy a new car; deciding which car to buy is again going to lead to stress. Buying a new home is very exciting but trying to decorate the home is stressful as well. So, good or bad, stress is any change in the environment that places new demands on our brains and bodies.

How can I Deal with Stressful Situations?

Stress affects all of us; each and every person in the world will experience stress. We cannot run away from stress but we can definitely learn to cope with it to the best of our ability. It is all a matter of taking control of our thoughts and actions when faced with stressful situations.

Let us look at a familiar situation where someone (we will call this person Mary) is stuck in traffic and running late for work. Let's say someone tries to pass by the side, and overtake Mary. The most common response to this kind of situation is that Mary gets angry at the other driver and shouts at him/her. Now, does that stop the other driver? Nope! Chances are that after overtaking Mary, the other driver might annoy her further, by shouting back at her or using offensive body language. The other driver still gets his way and Mary is left fretting about this all day. What could Mary have done in this situation? The first thing would be to relax since it is not in our hands to be able to control the traffic situation. Secondly, hey, use this time to think over things, spend those waiting moments actually relaxing and observing others. If you pass a smile at the person trying to pass you, it might bring a smile to the other person's face, this might actually let him/her let you get your way. So, you might emerge the winner in this situation. ☺

Stress in our lives is caused by both people and situations. The most important thing to do is to relax and understand the situation. I have practiced the following steps to deal with stressful situations and they have helped me to remain calm in many stress filled situations:

1) In preparing to deal with stress, an important first step should be to *accept the situation*; this leads to a sense of self-control. Okay, I am in this situation, what do I do to deal with it? Once we learn to control our thoughts, we are in a better state of mind than when we become nervous in a challenging environment.

2) The next step is to *accept our feelings* about the stressor, good or bad. These could be caused by people, situations, or events. When we are more focused, we can think of better ways to solve the problem.

3) The final step is to *relax the mind* and go into a meditative state. We need to use our mental powers to strengthen positive energies and eliminate negative thoughts. We can tame the mind to free itself of

distracting thoughts and emotions while in this state. If thoughts intrude and/or emotions arise, we should go through them, then come back to the relaxed state of mind by focusing on relaxing the mind. If the negative thoughts are overpowering, meditate a little more till you are in control, and can make decisions on how to approach the problem. If you still cannot focus, get up, move around, do something that pleases you; then come back again to meditate. Thinking in a relaxed state of mind leads to enhanced *problem solving and decision-making*. Once in a relaxed state of mind, you are in control of your thinking.

Exercising the brain by thinking good thoughts and visualizing goal attainment is a good way to release stress hormones and relax. When the brain is relaxed, it sends positive messages to the body that further calm the body. As we get into a meditative state and unwind our thoughts, we loosen up our tensed muscles making the flow of positive energy more directed towards positive outcomes. This leads to a feeling of goodness, a feeling that makes us happy and brings a smile to our faces.

Spheres of Stress

Change in any sphere of life can lead to stress. We deal with work, financial, emotional, environmental and health situations all the time. In trying to cope with the fast pace of life, we try to squeeze in whatever we can in a short period of time. I think what really helps, is slowing down a little, and organizing our work and time. Work organization and time management sets a routine for us. It is easier to cope when we know what comes next and are prepared to deal with it.

Some common examples of stress related to work, health, finance, emotions, society and environment can be:

Work: Driving to and from work, dealing with management and co-workers, receiving promotions or being passed for promotions, getting fired or laid off, attending meetings, meeting deadlines, etc.

Health: Minor health problems like tiredness, headaches, allergies, cold and cough, minor injuries, aches and pains; to dealing with chronic health problems, like surgery, hypertension, diabetes, hormonal problems and other illnesses.

Finance: Worrying about getting good jobs to earn enough money to pay bills – house rent, mortgage, auto loans, auto insurance, college tuition, medical bills, etc.

Emotions: Personal problems that effect relationships at home, work, and in the society.

Society: Trying to cope with the demands of family, work, friends and society, maintaining relationships, and social commitments.

Environment: The weather outside affects our internal bodies. Trying to adjust the body's thermostat to the outside climate is stressful to the mind and the body. What happens in the environment affects our perception and behavior.

Coping with Stress

If we learn to cope with stress and come up with ways that help reduce stress, we would be in a better position to deal with the stresses of life. Positive results can be achieved by learning new techniques and following them. For example:

- ❖ Be grateful for assets and accomplishments
- ❖ Circulate positive energy by keeping the environment clean and organized
- ❖ Eat nutritious food and reduce the quantity of food intake
- ❖ Exercise regularly, yogic exercises lead to relaxation and healing
- ❖ Laugh often, even when feeling low
- ❖ Regularly, take out time to do what we like doing
- ❖ Sleep for at least 7 hours a night; if possible, take power naps during the day.
- ❖ Socialize; spend time with people who make one feel good
- ❖ Think Positive, no matter what situation we are in

Note: To learn about stress management and relaxation techniques, please refer to chapters 6 to 10 that cover happy living techniques, breathing exercises, meditation, traditional and positive yoga in detail.

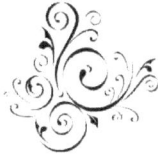

Chapter 4

RELAXATION AND STRESS MANAGEMENT FOR TEENS & YOUTH

Adopting the right attitude can convert a negative stress into a positive one.

- Hans Selye

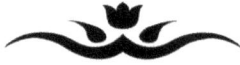

The greatest weapon against stress is our ability to choose one thought over another.

\- William James

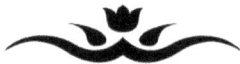

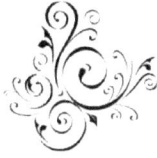

Today's youth, tomorrow's adults

I WILL LIVE MY LIFE TO THE FULLEST AND FIND MY PLACE IN THE WORLD

In order to develop our teens and youth into happy and peaceful adults, we have to instill in them the power of positive thinking, NOW. The seed of positivism we sow in them today, will yield the results in a few years when these teens hold the reigns in their hands.

Teens and youth today are faced with so many stresses that affect and disrupt their normal physical and psychological functioning and bring about changes in their thought and behavior processes. These stresses can be in any of the fields - psychological, emotional, physical, behavioral, health, school or family. As parents, we need to address stress related issues, in order to develop our teens into happy and successful adults with high self esteem.

Teens are very gullible and tend to give in to peer pressure in an effort to obtain a sense of belonging. Parents should instill good values in them and provide support and understanding so that they refrain from doing things that are not right for them. As parents, we need to guide our teens in the right direction so that they will grow up into happy and confident adults with high self esteem.

Stress in Teens and How It Affects Their Behavior

Psychological Negative thought processes - like focusing too much on negativity - decreases focus and concentration and may affect relationships and grades.

School Overload of schoolwork related to homework, after-school activities, and trying to cope with peer pressure may lead to missing assignments, low grades and low self esteem.

Family Family pressure in matters related to grades, social and cultural influence on teens, makes it very stressful for them to maintain a balance between family, peers and cultural demands.

Behavioral Family and emotional stresses can lead to behavioral adjustment problems related to changes in eating habits, increased aggressiveness, loss of interest in activities, and dependence on smoking and drinking.

Emotional Trying to cope with stressful activities can lead to anxiety, panic, mood swings, low self esteem, feelings of hopelessness, and loneliness.

Health Increased headaches, fatigue and vulnerability to stress and disease can arise when faced with stressful situations. These can further lead to digestive problems, weight gain, and insomnia.

Time Management

In a study on college students, it was found the students who perceived control of their time reported significantly greater evaluations of their performance, greater work and life satisfaction, less role ambiguity, less role overload, and fewer job-induced and somatic tensions (Macan, Shahani, Dipboye & Phillips).[1]

Results from a study examining self-care practices and perceived stress among psychology graduate students suggest that educating students about self-care practices can be an integral part of helping students manage stress associated with clinical training (Myers, Sweeney, Popick, Wesley, Bordfeld, & Fingerhut).[2]

Insomnia

Findings from a research study support a cognitive model of insomnia. Stress must be seen as a precipitating factor in the onset and maintenance of insomnia. Consequently, competencies to deal with dysfunctional sleep-related cognitions should be fostered in stress management programs. In turn, stress management should be a primary focus in the treatment of insomnia (Brand, Gerber, Pühse & Holsboer-Trachsler).[3]

Techniques to Deal with Stress

- ❖ Eat nutritious food
- ❖ Engage in fun activities
- ❖ Exercise regularly
- ❖ Get enough rest and sleep
- ❖ Think positive

HELPFUL TIPS – Start up

Simple Stress Reliever Techniques for Teens

Initial Steps

1. Consult a physician or counselor before starting on practicing any of the techniques mentioned.

2. Practice initially under the observance of an adult.

3. Have a positive attitude and belief in the positive outcome of the exercises.

4. Commit to setting out a fixed amount of time every day on a regular basis.

5. Try to practice at the same time every day.

Easy Steps

Consult physician → Adult Guidance → Positive Attitude → Commitment → Regular practice

HELPFUL TIPS
Simple Meditation Technique

Meditation is a process where you relax the mind and body by controlling your thoughts, giving the mind time to rest and rejuvenate. When we have a lot on our minds, it affects our focus and concentration. A few minutes spent on meditation everyday produce amazing results.

1. To begin meditation, sit comfortably in a relaxed position in a chair, or cross-legged on the floor.

2. Close your eyes and relax the facial muscles by emptying the brain of all thoughts and emotions. Bring a smile to the face. Relax.

3. Control your thoughts by relaxing the mind and giving it the time to enjoy the stillness. If thoughts keep intruding, relax and let the thoughts pass, then relax the mind again.

4. Focus, or visualize, on anything that makes you feel good about yourself and gears towards productivity.

5. Remain in this meditative and relaxed posture till you feel relaxed or for about 15-20 minutes. Meditate once a day for 10 minutes each in the morning and evening.

Easy Steps

Sit comfortably → Close eyes and relax face → Control the thoughts → Focus/visualize → Enjoy the meditation

HELPFUL TIPS
Simple Breathing Technique

Breathing exercises provide our bodies with the fuel it needs to run on. Just like we need gasoline in our cars to drive them, similarly, we need to regularly practice deep breathing exercises to repair our body and live a healthy life. When we inhale, we take in oxygen that cleanses our mind and body and clears the path for health and wellness. As we breathe in and concentrate on our breath, we relax our mind, which in turn relaxes our body.

Breathing Technique:

1. & 2. Repeat steps 1 and 2 as in the meditation technique.

3. Breathe in – Inhale through the nose, feel the oxygen travel into your lungs, your lungs will expand as the oxygen enters them and you will feel the chest expanding.

4. Hold the breath for five seconds.

5. Breathe out – Exhale through the nose or mouth, whatever you are comfortable with.

Do some breathing exercises when faced with challenging situations at school or home.

Easy Steps

Sit comfortably → Close eyes and relax face → Breathe in → Hold the breath → Breathe out

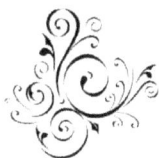

Chapter 5

EATING WISELY

It is all about **ME** *–* **M**indful **E**ating

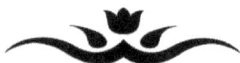

What I eat determines how I feel

the more heavy food I eat, the heavier I feel

Food is a cue that triggers the brain,

forgetting my health, I board the junk train

I need to promise myself that I will

NOT be a junkie for junk food,

I will TRAIN MY BRAIN to eat only food that

makes me feel good,

NOT the food that only looks good.

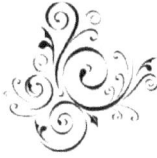

I am what I eat!

I WILL EAT TO PROVIDE ENERGY TO MY BODY, NOT TO ENJOY A FEW SECONDS OF TASTE

Some examples of diseases that can be healed to a great extent, even cured, by paying attention to eating healthy and nutritious food are hypertension, diabetes, allergies, and minor aches and pains. There is a lot of research that supports the effects of healthy eating in curing these illnesses. Many diseases can be controlled and healed to a large extent by controlling our eating.

HEALTH PROBLEM	FOODS TO AVOID
Hypertension	Salt, Fat, Carbohydrates, Sodium
Diabetes	Salt, Fat, Carbohydrates, Sodium, Sugar
Cholesterol	Salt, Fats, Carbohydrates, Sodium
Insomnia	Salt, Fats, Carbohydrates, Sodium

All the NO-NO foods contain toxins which get into our blood stream and affect our mental, emotional and physical well-being when they enter our bodies. When we eat too much fatty food, it slows down our focus and concentration, increasing irritability and anger, which further leads to lethargy and fatigue.

Growing up, I was always told that going to bed on a heavy stomach (full meal) leads to nightmares. As a child I did not pay much attention to that but now as an adult, I do agree with it. More often than not, I am very careful with my evening meals; I keep them light and have my dinner around 5:30 pm or so, and the night passes peacefully. Sometimes on weekends, when I eat a heavy meal, I can feel the effects of fatty food right away.

Eating fatty foods and carbohydrates for dinner or late at night might lead to

- ❖ discomfort throughout the night.
- ❖ disrupted sleep.
- ❖ getting up fatigued in the morning.
- ❖ puffed up face and eyes.
- ❖ weight gain.

The days I am careful with my eating, I sleep well, dream good and get up refreshed in the morning ready to deal with the challenges of the day.

Well, we all give in to cravings here and there and when we do, cleansing our system for a couple of days by eating fruits and vegetables provides immense relief to our brain and rest of the body organs and systems.

Our brains respond to certain cues in the environment and many times we give in to cravings. For example, the smell of food or an inviting sight of food, pulls us towards it and many times we eat even when we are full. This is the affect food has on us, it is a constant battle. Even when we try hard, we give in here and there.

Taking my own example, I normally eat fresh fruits and vegetables during weekdays when I am confined to my work space. Even at home, I am very good with sticking to my food schedule. But come weekends or a party at work, it is a big challenge for me not to eat that attractive, saliva-producing food. So, what is the solution here? It is difficult to control when you see all that food, your cravings try to win over you. Okay, sometimes we do give in to those cravings but cleansing our body for a couple of days after that helps. I am sharing with you what has helped me with my cravings:

1. Eat very small quantities of what is served and enjoy every bite of it. Try it, you will notice how just a couple of bites savored with conscious attention gives a satisfying feeling.

2. If I do give in to my cravings, I try not to feel guilty, instead I work on my craving by eating only fresh fruits and vegetables for the next couple of days.

3. I double up on my breathing exercises, yoga and meditation so that I can get back to my routine of self control.

Cleansing Our Bodies

Cleansing the body eliminates the toxins we take in when we eat excessive food to satisfy our cravings. I have personally tried a few detoxifying plans and they have worked wonders for me.

The best way to cleanse our system is to eat fresh fruits and vegetables. As the body is cleansed, one feels more energetic and also feels and looks better.

NOTE – Please consult a physician before starting on any plan.

COLORFUL FRUIT CLEANSE Mix and match to make fruit salads			
	DAY 1	**DAY 2**	**DAY 3**
Breakfast (9 am)	Apple (red)	Mango (yellow)	Papaya (orange)
Lunch (12 noon)	Grapes (green)	Kiwi (green)	Bananas (green)
Snack (3 pm)	Oranges (orange)	Blueberries (blue)	Strawberries (red)
Dinner (6 pm)	Cantaloupe (orange)	Watermelon (red)	Honeydew (green)

COLORFUL VEGETABLE CLEANSE

Mix and match to make salads and season   with salt, pepper and lime juice/vinegar

	DAY 1	DAY 2	DAY 3
Breakfast (9 am)	Pomegranate (red)	Avocado (green)	Beetroot (red)
Lunch (12 noon)	Corn (yellow)	Peppers (green, red, yellow, orange)	Cucumber (green)
Snack (3 pm)	Spinach/Kale (green)	Broccoli (green)	Onions (red)
Dinner (6 pm)	Tomatoes (red)	Watermelon (red)	Celery (green)

LIQIUDS FEEL-LIGHT PLAN

Mix and match fruit and veggies to make different smoothies, can add a little honey or sugar for sweet taste

	DAY 1	**DAY 2**	**DAY 3**
Breakfast (9 am)	**Apple, Banana and Strawberries Smoothie** (Blend apples, bananas, strawberries and 1% low fat organic milk)	**Papaya Shake** (Blend papayas, yogurt and 1% low fat organic milk)	Mango Shake (Blend mangoes, yogurt and 1% low fat organic milk)
Lunch (12 noon)	**Apple, Banana and Strawberries Smoothie**	**Papaya Shake**	Mango Shake
Snack (3 pm)	Tea/Coffee	Tea/Coffee	Tea/Coffee
Dinner (5 pm)	**Apple, Banana and Strawberries Smoothie**	**Papaya Shake**	Mango Shake

HEALTHY FOODS TO EAT REGULARLY

Almonds	Apples	Artichokes
Avocados	Bananas	Beet
Berries	Broccoli	Carrots
Cashews	Celery	Cucumbers
Garlic	Ginger	Grapes
Guavas	Olives	Pears
Peppers	Pineapple	Pomegranate
Pumpkin	Tomatoes	Walnuts
Whole Grains	Yogurt	Zucchini

HELPFUL TIPS FOR SIMPLE EATING

RULES TO FOLLOW DAILY

Benefits:

What happens when we see attractive food in front of us? Even though we might be full, we are tempted to eat it. Food is a cue to the brain. From past experience, the brain has been trained to eat when we see food. We need to be able to control our brain and teach our brain new techniques to refrain from food that is not good for us. Once we start practicing these new techniques, they become a habit. The essential thing here is to follow this new technique for at least a month so that it becomes a habit. Making these simple techniques an everyday habit will lead to a healthy life and make one feel good and look good. The body feels light when we eat light nutritious food; eating fats and carbohydrates leads to extra stress on our digestive system. The following techniques have helped me a lot and I would like to share them with you.

1. **Eat five small meals a day – breakfast, morning snack, lunch, afternoon snack and dinner**. Keep in mind the quotes – have breakfast for yourself, share lunch with a friend and leave dinner for the enemy; eat breakfast like a king, lunch like a commoner and dinner like a pauper.

2. **Breakfast should be a little heavier than the other meals -** There is quite a few hours of gap between dinner and breakfast. *Break-fast* is essential as you are *breaking a fast of 7-8 hours;* you need the energy to start the day. A quick smoothie made with apples, bananas and 1% low fat organic milk provides the nutrients and energy needed to begin the day. Salad for lunch with a little fruit and a small piece of wholegrain bread; a small

200 calories meal for dinner eaten at least three hours before going to bed; and light snacks (fruit, vegetable, juice, health bar, almonds, raisins) as morning and evening snacks, give us the nutrients and energy for maintaining a healthy brain and body.

3. **Drink plenty of water** – Water cleanses our body, the more we drink it, the more toxins are flushed out of the body. It is essential to drink at least eight glasses of water every day. To make it a habit, set regular times to drink water, that way you don't forget.

4. **Enjoy what you eat** – If you really crave a food, take a bite and let the food linger in the mouth, enjoying its taste to the fullest. Even a couple of bites of your favorite food, if savored and enjoyed, will lead to a satisfied feeling and decrease cravings. Do not deprive yourself but reduce the quantity considerably. Remember – we eat to provide energy to the body.

5. **Eat more of fresh fruits and vegetables** – Fresh fruit and vegetables are the best; they can also be consumed in juice form.

6. **Chew the food** – Eat small quantities of food at one time and chew the food for a while before swallowing it so that the body can use all the nutrients and transform the food into energy.

7. **Eat only when hungry** – Do not eat if you are full from the previous meal.

<u>Easy Steps</u>

SIMPLE EATING HABITS → To move
forward (**FWD**) in healthful living → Avoid
foods made with **F**at, **W**heat, **D**airy→ HAPPY
HEALTHY LIFE

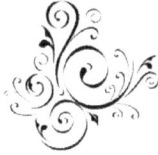

Chapter 6

HAPPY LIVING

TECHNIQUES AND STRATEGIES

The air we breathe, the water we drink, and the land we inhabit are not only critical elements in the quality of life we enjoy – they are a reflection of the majesty of our Creator.

- Rick Perry

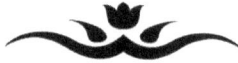

1. *Breathing Exercises*
2. *Chanting*
3. *Fresh Fruit and Vegetable Meals*
4. *Face, Hair and Full Body Massage*
5. *Foot Exercises*
6. *Hand Exercises*
7. *Meditation and Relaxation*
8. *Music Therapy*
9. *Self-talk for Motivation*
10. *Yoga – Traditional*
11. *Yoga – Positive*

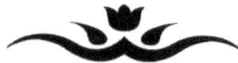

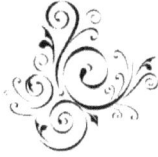

TECHNIQUES TO ACHIEVE OPTIMAL WELLNESS

Faith and commitment are the two most important ingredients in the recipe for success. Spending a couple of hours daily on ourselves can lead to amazing results. I personally practice the following techniques on a regular basis. I must say that acceptance, positive thinking and being happy no matter what, has helped me immensely in dealing with the stress in my life. I am grateful for all the stress in life because if it weren't for this stress, I would not be the grateful person I am today. I religiously practice the following techniques and consider them as great remedies for relaxation and stress relief.

1. **Breathing Exercises:**

Oxygen is life force, the more we breathe in oxygen, the better our health will be. I have personally lost a lot of weight by doing breathing exercises only. I committed myself to doing at last 30 minutes of breathing exercises for a couple of months and was amazed with the results! By continuing these exercises for a few more months, I lost about 50 pounds.

Please refer to the exercises mentioned in the chapter on Breathing for more details on breathing exercises.

2. Chanting:

Repeating uplifting and motivating words while sitting in a relaxing meditative posture calms the mind and increases focus and concentration. For example, when I feel hurt in relationships, I start chanting uplifting words about my enduring relationship with the positive energy in the universe. Doing this gives me my strength back and makes me emotionally strong.

3. Fresh Fruit and Vegetable Meals:

Eating fresh fruit and vegetables most of the time cleanses our body internally and externally, clears the body of toxins and brings a glow to the face.

Please refer to the chapter on Nutrition for diet plans that are easy to follow.

4. Face, Hair and Full Body Massage:

Massage has a very soothing effect and invigorates us mentally and physically. Massaging the face in circular motions using a face lotion brings a glow to the face and makes one look younger. Start by massaging at the forehead, areas around the eyes, nose, cheeks, and ears; end by massaging the chin and area around the lips. The same affect is seen when the scalp is massaged with oil. Massage in circular motions with the fingertips starting at the hairline and going back all the way to the nape. Massaging the whole body with warm oil before taking a shower rejuvenates the body internally and gives it an external glow as well.

5. **Foot Exercises:**

    Our feet carry us around all day long, foot exercises provide relaxation to the feet and the whole body. A simple foot exercise can be done while sitting on the bed or on the floor. Sit comfortably, bring your legs together, feet upright touching each other. Rotate the feet together slowly clockwise ten times, then anti-clockwise ten times. After the rotations, point the toes away from the body and curl the soles of the feet. Enjoy the relaxed feeling!

6. **Hand Exercises:**

    While our feet carry the weight of the body, our hands help us perform our chores and lift weights. Hand exercises keep our hands strong. Sit in a comfortable position and concentrate on the hands. Start with forming a fist with your hand, then open the hand, stretching the palms and fingers as much as you can. Repeat open-close movement a few times with both hands. This exercise can be done with one hand at a time or with both hands simultaneously. Enjoy the feeling of relaxation as you stretch the palms of your hands!

7. **Meditation and Relaxation:**

    Our brains do the most work. They perceive stimuli in the environment, receive the neural information and transmit that information to the rest of our body. Our physical health depends on our mental health. It is essential to relax the brain by doing meditation regularly. When the brain is relaxed, it is in a better state to guide us toward positivism. Meditation involves relaxing our brain by relieving it of all stressful thoughts. A simple process like just concentrating on the breath for a few moments has tremendous beneficial effects.

Please refer to the techniques mentioned in the chapter on Meditation to learn more about relaxation techniques.

8. **Music Therapy:**

   Music has no language. Listening to music soothes and strengthens our cognitive abilities. Listening to any kind of music can have a soothing effect on our emotional self. No matter what the beat or rhythm, music relaxes the brain and enhances cognitive functioning. When our cognitive abilities are strengthened, we are more in control of ourselves to be optimistic and look at the positive side of whatever goes on in our lives. In addition to improving our mental and physical health, music positively influences our personal, emotional and social well being. Relaxation improves our communication skills, which further strengthen our relationships.

9. **Self-talk for Motivation:**

   Talking to ourselves sometimes helps us to look at things in a different perspective. Many times when I am distressed, I talk to myself. Most of the time when I talk to myself, I am made aware by my own thinking of how I have dealt with a situation, what I have done to improve that situation and what I should have done or can do now to resolve the problem related to that situation. This thinking motivates me to accept the situation and deal with stress to the best of my ability. All it takes is to look at the positive in every situation and work on improving what is in my control. Self-talk gears me into action.

10. Yoga (Traditional):

I constantly practice traditional and positive yoga exercises which help me relax and work toward achieving happiness by thinking positive. Regular practice of yoga techniques enhances mental, physical and spiritual well-being.

Please refer to the techniques mentioned in the chapter on traditional Yoga to learn more about traditional yoga postures.

11. Yoga (Positive):

While practicing traditional yoga postures, I realized that I felt more relaxed and energized when I smiled and was happy while practicing yoga. This, in turn, helped me to connect to the positive energy around me while visualizing beneficial outcomes. It seemed like I reaped double the benefits when I visualized positive results of what I wanted to achieve. This also took me deep into relaxation, leading to an elated feeling of connection to the universe. All this experience motivated me to come up with something I could practice regularly, was easy to remember in steps, and follow accordingly. I named these innovative techniques POSITIVE YOGA. Positive yoga emphasizes concentrating on positive thoughts and visualizing fulfilling results. It is a combination of yoga postures which include a relaxed posture, breathing oxygen exercises, smiling to be happy, visualizing positive outcomes, thinking of what is going on in our life and how we can improve things. Once we have relaxed our thoughts, we can connect to the energy flow around us and bring the positive energy towards ourselves to get a feeling of contentment.

Positive Yoga follows *eight* steps which are practiced in a flow. Each of the eight steps need to be given individual attention to reap the best benefits of positive yoga as described below.

Posture - Sit/lie down in a comfortable position

Oxygen - Inhale the life force, oxygen and feel refreshed

Smile - Be happy and exercise the facial muscles

Introspect - Turn your thoughts inwards

Transcend - Rise above the situation, surpass, exceed

Integrate – Illuminate and provide light within

Visualize – Think about positive outcomes and success

Energize – Enjoy the energized feeling!

The chapter on Positive Yoga has innovative wellness techniques which are a combination of modified traditional breathing techniques and yoga postures, in addition to guided imagery and positive energy.

Note: Each of the above techniques have their own benefits and can be practiced anywhere depending on how you feel, where you are, and the time you have available.

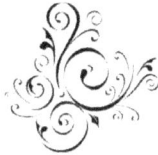

Chapter 7

BREATHING EXERCISES FOR HEALTHY LIVING

"Breath is the bridge which connects life to consciousness, which unites your body to your thoughts."

- Thich Nhat Hanh

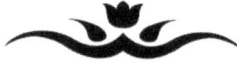

"How do you tell if something's alive? You check for breathing."
- Markus Zusak, The Book Thief

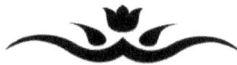

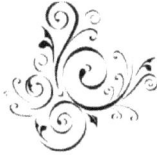

The importance of OXYGEN

Breath is life. When we inhale oxygen, it rejuvenates the brain cells and increases our energy levels, which, in turn, send positive messages to the entire body thereby enhancing positive thought processes. Oxygen plays a vital role in maintaining and revitalizing the body's vital organs and the digestive, nervous, circulatory, and respiratory systems. It purifies the blood and removes toxins circulating in our blood systems.

Breathing exercises have been found to be very helpful in losing weight, managing stress, and improving and maintaining overall health. In this book, I am sharing with you some breathing exercises which helped me lose weight and maintain it. Motivated with my weight loss and how it changed my life mentally, physically and spiritually, I started concentrating on Happiness, Wellness and Positive Thinking (HWP). These terms are the very basis of the innovative techniques I have used to come up with positive yoga, breathing exercises, and meditation techniques. The techniques are very short and simple but what is required to achieve results is regularity, commitment, and persistence. The exercises can be performed by sitting on a chair or cross-legged on the floor. You can also practice these by lying down on the floor or bed. Yoga breathing exercises, termed "Pranayama," help deal with chronic illnesses like hypertension, cholesterol, heart problems, diabetes, and various other day-to-day problems, which can be dealt with by making lifestyle changes. Breathing exercises help tremendously to relax and reduce stress. Taking a few deep breaths when stressed, relaxes and prepares for the coming challenges. If you don't have time to do other kinds of exercise, just doing the breathing exercises will give the benefits of other forms of exercise. What a great feeling it is when you are relaxed. A relaxed state of mind leads to better mental, physical, spiritual, emotional and intellectual functioning.

Breathing Exercises and Stress Management

Breathing exercises have been my savior. Whenever I have been in stress, be it related to weight gain problems, relationships or financial setbacks, the best way I deal with stress is to intensify my routine of breathing and meditation. When I am stressed, I increase the time I spend on my breathing exercises and meditation. This not only helps me with dealing with that particular stress causing event, but also takes me a step forward in discovering myself. Every time I go back to increasing my breathing and meditation practice, I see a new me, geared to lead a meaningful and purposeful life.

Breathing Exercises and Weight Management

Till a few years ago, I had always been overweight. I was pleasantly fat as a teenager, but as the years went by, I kept adding on weight. Finally, around the year 2002, I read about how breathing exercises help with weight loss. I challenged myself to do half-an-hour breathing exercises every day for two months. That was my first success with weight loss. As time went by, I was motivated to add yoga exercises to my routine and that was the ultimate success in losing weight. I lost over 80 pounds. Motivated with my success, I got certified as a yoga instructor and wellness consultant. Over the years, I have developed some new yoga postures and via this book, I would like to share some ancient breathing exercises, yoga postures, and meditation techniques, in addition to the new POSITIVE YOGA breathing exercises, yoga postures, and meditation techniques I have developed. These techniques have helped me to maintain good mental and physical health, and lead a life filled with positive thoughts and happiness.

Benefits of Breathing Exercises

❖ Achieve a relaxed state of mind by refining inner thoughts

❖ Channel positive energy to achieve optimal wellness

❖ Cleanse and relax the mind

❖ Enhance positivism by controlling thought flow towards desired goals

❖ Improve focus and concentration

❖ Improve overall health

❖ Increase the flow of positive energy inside the body and around us in the environment

❖ Manage stress and relax the mind

❖ Recharge mentally, physically and spiritually

❖ Release stress and calm the nervous system

❖ Triumph over daily hassles

Breathing Techniques for Optimal Health

OM (AUM) BREATHING

"Om" or "Aum" breathing technique is a very old yoga breathing exercise. If practiced consistently, it has lasting beneficial effects on our overall health.

Step-by-Step Instructions:

1. Sit comfortably in a chair, or cross-legged on the floor, with the spine elongated. Relax the mind by emptying it of all thoughts and emotions. Focus on the breath.

2. Inhale by taking a deep breath through the nose, expanding the chest, diaphragm and upper abdomen, as you inhale oxygen into your lungs.

3. Exhale, contracting the stomach muscles and drawing them towards the spine. As you exhale, say the word "aum" or "om", for as long as possible. Start the exhale, saying "O (A)..." as you begin to exhale and end with "...M" as you end with the exhalation.

4. Repeat the "inhale-exhale" a few times or till you are deeply involved in the process.

5. To begin, do 5 repetitions and take it to 15-20 or whatever you are comfortable with as you progress.

SKULL BREATHING
Kapalbhati

1. This breathing exercise can be done by sitting cross-legged on the floor or bed, or sitting on a chair with the spine straight. Place hands on the knees with palms facing upwards, thumb and index finger tips meeting. Relax the mind and body.

2. Inhale by taking a deep breath.

3. As you exhale, contract the stomach muscles by drawing them forcefully toward the spine. Expel the air out with a forceful and audible blow through the nose.

4. Repeat the process in steps 2 and 3 in succession till you get into the flow of inhale-exhale. Keep in mind, all the breathing is done through the nose.

5. Start with 10 repetitions and take it all the way to 100 slowly.

<u>Easy Steps</u>

Inhale through the nose

↓

Contract stomach muscles as you exhale

↓

Blow air out through the nose

↓

Get into the flow of inhale-exhale

ALTERNATE NOSTRIL BREATHING
Anulom-Vilom

1. Sit comfortably in a relaxed position, head and back aligned, cross-legged on the floor, or on a chair.

2. Relax and empty the mind of all thoughts and emotions. Concentrate on your relaxed mental, physical and spiritual calmness.

3. Bring your right hand up to the nose and press the right nostril with your thumb. Keep the rest of the hand straight, with palms facing outwards and fingers pointing upwards.

4. Breathe in deeply from the left nostril; hold the breath for a few seconds and clip both nostrils by pressing the left nostril with the right ring finger.

5. Keeping the left nostril pressed with the right ring finger, release the thumb from the right nostril and exhale.

6. Relax a couple of seconds, then start inhaling through the right nostril.

7. Bring the thumb back to press the right nostril, again clipping the nostrils with the thumb and ring finger.

8. Release the ring finger from the left nostril and breathe out.

9. This completes one cycle of Anulom-Vilom.

10. Repeat five to ten cycles with the same hand or by alternating hands.

ALTERNATE NOSTRIL BREATHING (continued)

<u>Easy Steps</u>

Press right nostril with thumb; inhale through the left
nostril

↓

Clip nostrils with thumb on right and ring on left nostril,
respectively

↓

Release thumb from right nostril; exhale

↓

Inhale through right nostril; clip nostrils again

↓

Release left nostril; exhale

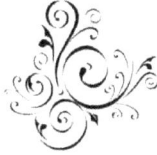

Chapter 8

MEDITATION PRACTICES FOR POSITIVE THINKING

Health is the greatest gift, contentment the greatest wealth, faithfulness the best relationship.

\- Buddha

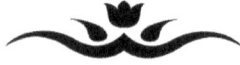

*Prayer is when you talk to God; meditation
is when you listen to God.*

\- Diana Robinson

*Meditation brings wisdom; lack of mediation leaves
ignorance. Know well what leads you forward and
what hold you back, and choose the path that leads to
wisdom.*

\- Buddha

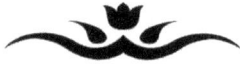

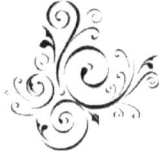

Relax, think positive and meditate to be happy!

To achieve a happy and meaningful life, it is important to look into and work on improving ourselves. Like Mahatma Gandhi said:

Be the change you wish to see in the world.

Since we can control our minds and thoughts, the best thing to do in stressful situations is to look into ourselves. As an example, let us look at how we sometimes frantically look for something we have misplaced. After looking for it for a while and not finding it, if we quietly sit down and focus just on where it could be, then more often than not, we normally get an insight into where the thing could be. What else is this but meditation?

Life is fast-paced and often becomes hectic when we try to cope with its demands. In an attempt to meet all the demands, we rely heavily on our brain and the rest of the body. The brain and heart over exert to help us achieve our needs. Our mind is never at rest. Our bodies do get a little relief when we sleep but our mind is still in an active mode as we dream when we are asleep. It therefore becomes very important that our brain gets some rest to calm down, and become more focused. The best way to do this is to relax the brain by meditating. Meditation helps to relax our mind by helping us concentrate on the positive thoughts while taking us away from negative ones. With regular practice, we can bring positive energy towards ourselves by always thinking positive and diverting negative thoughts away. Once we have attained inner peace and serenity, our mind will stay in a state of blissful happiness, which is the root of mental, physical and spiritual well-being.

Meditation is a technique in which the mind is focused on a relaxing thought, object or just quietness. The whole attention is diverted towards that thought or object leading to more focus and concentration and achieving a relaxed state of mind. Performing simple rituals like becoming aware of our breath, listening to music, visualizing something, and chanting a mantra, are all examples of meditation. When we meditate, the thought processes cease and the mind calms down, leading to achievement of a state of liberation and experience of inner happiness.

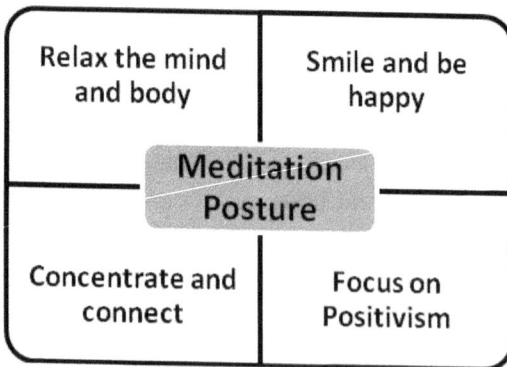

Relax the mind and body	Smile and be happy
Meditation Posture	
Concentrate and connect	Focus on Positivism

__Benefits of Meditation__

- ❖ Build positive self concept
- ❖ Build self confidence
- ❖ Control brain functions and mental thought processes
- ❖ Enhance immune system by releasing good hormones
- ❖ Experience inner peace
- ❖ Healthy shiny skin
- ❖ Improve family, peer, social and work relationships
- ❖ Improve focus and concentration
- ❖ Increase creativity
- ❖ Increase memory
- ❖ Increase orderliness and organization
- ❖ Increase strength and productivity
- ❖ Normalize blood pressure, cholesterol and sugar levels
- ❖ Pain management
- ❖ Perceive positive stimuli
- ❖ Reach deeper levels of relaxation
- ❖ Reduce allergies and viral infections
- ❖ Reduce anxiety and increase confidence
- ❖ Reduce need for medical help and care
- ❖ Release stress and tension
- ❖ Reverse the aging process

Common Meditation Techniques

Keeping the benefits of meditation in mind, sit comfortably in a relaxed state of mind and focus on your breathing. Feel and enjoy the positive energy as you breathe in and retain the breath. Relax as you breathe out.

Chanting Meditation: Pick up any word or phrase you like and chant it at a comfortable pace. Some commonly used words are: "Om," peace, love, happiness, faith, etc.

Counting Meditation: Seated in a comfortable position, breathe in to a slow count of ten, hold the breath to another count of ten, and exhale to a count of ten.

Focus Meditation: Focus your gaze on an object, e.g. a candle, a nice picture or a bare wall. Breathe in, hold and breathe out, keeping your gaze focused on the object.

Music Meditation: Listen to soothing music, like the flute, and relax.

Visual Meditation: Visualize an object or scene that gives you peace and makes you happy. Sit in a comfortable posture. Focus on the breath as you breathe in, visualize the happy thought and feel the positive energy flow through the body, focus on the breath as you breathe out.

NOTE – All the meditation techniques require relaxing the mind along with focus and concentration. As a beginner, start with meditating for about 5 minutes or so. Gradually increase meditation time to 15 or 20 minutes. These techniques can also be practiced for 3 to 5 times a day for shorter time periods. The best time to practice seems to be early morning as the mind is fresh and relaxed after a few hours of resting.

IMPORTANT POINTS TO KEEP IN MIND WHILE PRACTICING MEDITATION

Meditation Posture - Sit in a comfortable position, either on a chair or cross legged on the floor. The hands can rest in your lap or kept on the knees with the palms facing upwards and the forefinger and thumb touching. Meditation can also be practiced by lying down on the bed or floor. The main thing to keep in mind is that the back should be straight and there should be a smile on the face.

Relax the mind and body - Close the eyes, empty the mind of all thoughts and emotions, smile and focus on the breath. Maintain a relaxed state of mind by concentrating on positive thoughts and diverting negative thoughts away from the mind. If an unwanted thought keeps bothering you by coming back, let it take its course and then revert back to positive thinking. With practice, you will be able to empty your mind and concentrate on the positivism around you.

Concentrate and connect - Once the state of relaxation has been achieved, concentrate on your breath, visualize something, listen to a sound, repeat a positive word or just try to connect to the silence around you. Just sitting in silence and connecting to the positive energy in the universe is very refreshing.

Focus on positivism - If something is really bothering you, it becomes difficult to focus. In this case, once you are totally relaxed and are concentrating, divert your thoughts to visualize the positive outcomes of the situation or feeling that is bothering you. If you are working on healing a particular part of your body, feel the positive energy travel to that area and feel the area being healed; this is very important. When we imagine the healing, we feel happy and good hormones are released in our body that enhance healing.

Smile and be happy - Once fully engaged in the meditation process, one attains satisfaction and fulfillment. A new happier individual emerges. Bask in the elated feeling of happiness once the connection to the universal positive energy, which fills you with positive emotions, is established. As you come out of the meditative state, keep the smile on your face and bow down in gratefulness with folded hands. Smile as you go in, go through and come out of the meditation process.

Think positive, be happy and be at peace with yourself and the outside world. Enjoy!

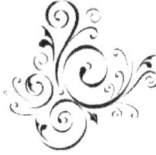

Chapter 9

TRADITIONAL YOGA FOR MIND-BODY RELAXATION

Yoga teaches us to cure what need not be endured and endure what cannot be cured.

- B.K.S. Iyengar

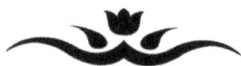

You

Obtain

Great

Achievement

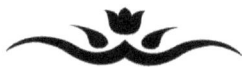

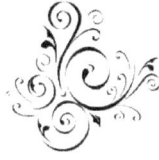

Think positive, practice YOGA and heal!

Yoga is an ancient philosophical discipline which teaches us to harmonize the mind, body and soul. Practicing yoga exercises regularly cleanses and massages the internal and external body, Yoga practice helps us to lead a more fulfilling, satisfying, healthy, and stress-free life. On a physical level, yoga builds strength and vitality, massages the internal organs and strengthens the digestive, circulatory and immune systems thereby enhancing well-being. For the mind, it improves memory and concentration, sharpens the intellect, increases emotional intelligence and steadies the emotions to achieve a richer and more fulfilling life. On a deeper spiritual level, the practice of yoga leads to self-awareness and increases connection to the universal positive energy. Practice of yoga strengthens the mind, body and spirit, and helps prevent major illnesses. It helps to cure and deal with common health problems like allergies, blood pressure, cholesterol, diabetes, stress management and weight loss.

<u>Benefits of Yoga</u>

- ❖ Calm the mind and body
- ❖ Cleanse, massage and nourish all body organs
- ❖ Create a sense of inner peace and well being
- ❖ Detoxify the body completely
- ❖ Enhance digestion
- ❖ Fight depression
- ❖ Improve concentration and decision making
- ❖ Improve muscle tone
- ❖ Improve posture
- ❖ Improve sleep
- ❖ Increase energy levels and stamina
- ❖ Lower blood pressure and cholesterol levels
- ❖ Pain management and prevention
- ❖ Release stress
- ❖ Strengthen the immune system
- ❖ Weight loss and management

Remember: Think positive, be happy, and be at peace

with yourself.

Common Types of Yoga Sessions

Yoga has spread and segmented into various types of yoga practices that address specific ailments and stress-related illnesses. Some of the most popular yoga sessions are:

❖ Breathing Yoga
❖ Chair Yoga
❖ Children and Teen Yoga
❖ Heart Healthy Yoga
❖ Invigorating Yoga
❖ Laughter Yoga
❖ Meditation Yoga
❖ Prenatal and Postnatal Yoga
❖ Restorative Yoga
❖ Women Yoga
❖ Yoga for Allergies and Asthma
❖ Yoga for Digestion
❖ Yoga for Happy Living
❖ Yoga for Heart Health
❖ Yoga for Hypertension
❖ Yoga to Improve Circulation
❖ Yoga for Insomnia
❖ Yoga for Positive Thinking
❖ Yoga for Spinal Alignment
❖ Yoga for Stress Management
❖ Yoga for Weight Loss
❖ … and so on

SIDDHASANA
Perfect Posture
Siddh = Perfect; *Asana* = Posture

Benefits:

- ✓ Decreases stiffness in hip, knee and ankle joints
- ✓ Enhances spiritual connection
- ✓ Helpful for people suffering from asthma, hypertension, insomnia and weight problems
- ✓ Helps in balancing blood pressure
- ✓ Helps in concentrating and relaxing the mind
- ✓ Improves memory and digestion
- ✓ Stimulates the brain; relaxes and calms the nervous system

Step-by-Step Instructions:

1. Sit on the floor in a comfortable position with both legs stretched out, arms on the sides of the body with hands touching the floor, palms facing downwards.

2. Slowly bend the left leg at the knee and slide it into the groin. Place the left heel against the perineum, the area just below the reproductive organs or the area between the genital organs and theanus.

3. Repeat this with the right leg placing the right foot on top of the left foot against the pubic bone, area just above the genitals. Turn the sole of right foot upward and tuck the toe in front of the left foot. The heels should be one above the other and the ankles should be touching.

4. Place hand on thighs with palms facing upwards, the thumb and forefinger lightly touching each other and the other three fingers extended.

5. Sit in this position with eyes closed, spine erect, holding the pose till you feel comfortable.

DANDASANA
Staff Posture
Dand = Stick; *Asana* = Posture

Benefits:

- ✓ Improves digestion and tones kidneys
- ✓ Improves sitting posture and spinal alignment
- ✓ Relaxes the feet by stretching the feet muscles
- ✓ Stretches the shoulder, chest and back muscles
- ✓ Strengthens thigh and leg muscles

Step-by-Step Instructions:

1. Sit on the floor with legs extended straight in front of you, spine erect and hands on the floor besides the hips, palms facing downward and gently pressing into the ground. Beginners can rest their back against the wall with the shoulder blades touching the walls.

2. Tighten the thigh muscles rotating them inwards and pressing them down to the floor.

3. The feet should be vertical, flexed and parallel to each other.

4. Stretch the spine upward imagining the spine to be a stick, keeping the back and head aligned.

5. Relax the neck and shoulders; drop the shoulder blades down the back so that they rotate towards each other.

Sit in this position for a minute or so.

VAJRASANA
Thunderbolt or Diamond Posture
Vajra = Thunderbolt or diamond; *Asana* = Posture

Benefits:

✓ Aids in digestive processes and gastric problems, helps to lose weight
✓ Increases secretion from glands
✓ Relaxes the mind and increases concentration and focus
✓ Relieves knee pain, strengthens thighs and calf muscles

Step-by-Step Instructions:

1. Stand straight and slowly come down to a kneeling position with the toes pointing away from the body.

2. Sit back on the heels.

3. Straighten the spine and sit with hands resting on the thighs, palms facing downwards. Balance weight on both legs.

4. Look in front and slowly close the eyes. Breathe normally through the nose. Sit in this position for as long as it is comfortable.

5. Return to the original position.

BADDHAKONASANA
Cobbler's Posture
Baddha = **Bound,** *Kona* = **Angle;** *Asana* = **Posture**

Benefits:

- ✓ Decreases depression and anxiety
- ✓ Good pose to practice and prepare to ease childbirth
- ✓ Helps relieve symptoms of menstrual periods and menopause
- ✓ Reduces fat from the thighs, especially stretching the inner thighs
- ✓ Stimulates the abdominal and reproductive organs, therapeutic for fertility
- ✓ Stimulates the heart and circulatory system

Step-by-Step Instructions:

1. Sit with legs extended straight out in front of you. Exhale, slowly bend the knees and bring the heels of both the feet toward the pelvis. Press the soles of the feet together and drop the knees out to the sides.

2. Sit up straight, pressing the heels as close to the pelvis as is comfortable. Grasp each toe with hands pressing the outer edges of the feet firmly into the ground.

3. Breathe normally.

4. Sit in this position for a few minutes or till comfortable.

5. Take a deep breath and slowly stretch out legs to come back to the original position.

MAKARASANA
Crocodile Posture
Makra = **Crocodile;** *Asana* = **Posture**

Benefits:

- ✓ Beneficial for asthma and allergy problems
- ✓ Helps reduce blood pressure
- ✓ Relaxes the whole body from head to toe
- ✓ Relieves stress and enhances relaxation
- ✓ Stretches the neck and chest

Step-by-Step Instructions:

1. Lie down on the floor, face down and resting the forehead on the floor, arms on the sides, hands by the sides of the thighs, legs straight, and chest touching the ground.

2. Slowly bring the arms to the front and stretch them outwards, fingers pointing away from the body.

3. Lengthen both legs so that the toes are pointing out. Relax all the body muscles and enjoy the stretch. Feel the body weight supported by the floor.

4. Stay in this position for a couple of minutes or as long as it is comfortable.

5. To release, bring the arms back to the sides and come back to the original prone position.

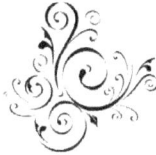

Chapter 10

BEAUTY LIES WITHIN US - POSITIVE YOGA

A man is but the product of his thoughts; what he thinks, he becomes.

- Mahatma Gandhi

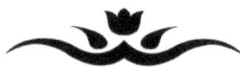

Posture

Oxygen

Smile

Introspect

Transcend

Integrate

Visualize

Energize

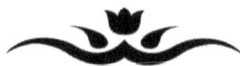

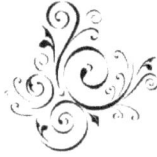

Positive Yoga Techniques

Positive yoga is a combination of innovative relaxing postures and popular yoga postures. Many people view yoga as turning and twisting their bodies to achieve certain postures. The more important factor of yoga is the ability to inhale oxygen, retain the breath, and exhale the toxins out of the body. What is important while doing yoga is your state of mind. It is imperative to concentrate on the breath and think positive while doing yoga or any other exercise. You will gain double the benefits if your mind is into it.

Important points to keep in mind while doing positive yoga:

1. Breathing techniques are important while doing yoga.

2. You normally do the inhaling when the body is stretched and exhale while bending over in a posture.

3. Relax the face and mind while performing yoga.

4. Think positive and be happy for putting in the effort to deal with problems.

5. Focus on the problem area and visualize its healing; keeping the eyes closed helps to focus more.

POSITIVE YOGA WELLNESS TECHNIQUES

Positive Wellness exercises are a variation of the ancient breathing techniques, which help in dealing with today's fast-paced life and the stress that comes with it. By focusing on the event/situation that causes the stress, called "stressor," and visualizing positive thoughts and outcomes, one can deal with the situation in a more effective way. Being optimistic leads to positivism and directs the flow of energy in the desired direction. It involves *five* steps:

1. **Relax**: Sit comfortably cross-legged or on a chair in a relaxed position. Align the head, back and spine. Relax the brain and body as you begin with the breathing exercises.

2. **Inhale**: Take a deep breath, feel the lungs, chest, diaphragm and upper abdomen expand as the oxygen travels through them.

3. **Think Positive**: Focus on positive thoughts that come to your mind and let the negative thoughts pass. Be optimistic and feel happy for repaying your body for all the effort it puts in for you.

4. **Be Happy**: Concentrate and visualize achieving your goals. Keeping the eyes closed helps increase focus and channel positive energy and oxygen towards the goal.

5. **Exhale**: To exhale, breathe out by pressing the abdomen towards the spine and expelling all the air out like forcing air out of a balloon.

<u>Benefits of Positive Yoga</u>

- ❖ Enhances mind-body connection by relaxing the mind, spine and entire body
- ❖ Facilitates digestion and provides relief from gastric pain.
- ❖ Good starting and ending relaxing posture for yoga exercise, meditation and pranayama
- ❖ Helps to lose weight and maintain weight, especially in the hips and thigh areas
- ❖ Improves spinal alignment, posture and body balance
- ❖ Increases concentration and focus; relieves stress, tension, anxiety and fatigue
- ❖ Relaxes the facial muscles and brings a glow to the face
- ❖ Relieves knee pain, strengthens thighs and calf muscles
- ❖ Relieves stress, tension, anxiety and fatigue
- ❖ Stretches the spine, strengthens the shoulders, arms, elbows, wrists, hands and fingers

POSITIVE YOGA
BREATHE-MEDITATE TECHNIQUE

This innovative technique gives double benefits of breathing and meditation. Practice it every day to enjoy the benefits of optimal wellness. It cleanses the brain and paves the way for the flow of positive energy through the mind-body pathways. Practice this exercise when you are stressed out or in a state of internal turmoil. This technique also helps to control emotions; sleep better and improve digestion. It increases the ability to face disturbing stimulators and win over them. When you are at peace with yourself, you will bring peace towards you. This exercise will benefit anyone and everyone.

1. This breathing exercise should be done in a position that makes you feel very comfortable. You can sit on the floor, bed or chair, spine elongated. Relax the mind and body.

2. Bring a broad smile to your face, keeping your lips pursed. This way you exercise the muscles around your mouth, which helps reduce the fine lines that come to the lips and the area around the lips with age. As you smile, good hormones travel in the body, directing positive energy throughout your body and giving you the glow of happiness.

3. Inhale, and feel the life-force, oxygen, and vital positive energy, traveling to the brain showering positivism.

4. Breathe normally, visualize the life-force, oxygen, moving from the brain to the rest of your body, purifying and filling it with radiant energy, traveling through your body in the following sequence: forehead, face, throat, chest, upper abdomen, lower

abdomen, pelvic area, legs, and finally moving to the arms. Enjoy the feeling!

5. Fold your hands in prayer position, and bow your head in gratefulness.

<u>Easy Steps</u>

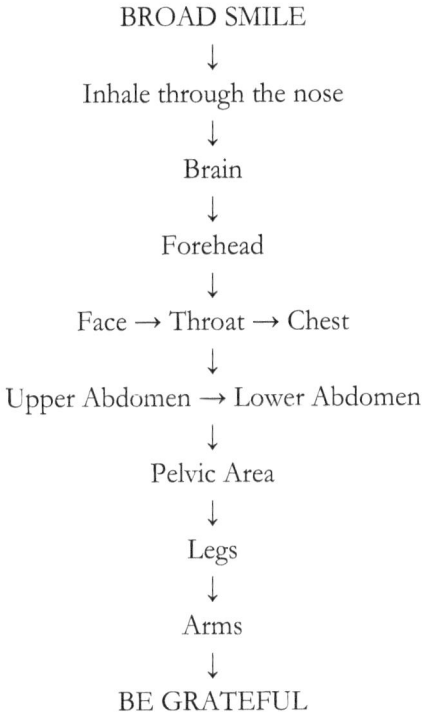

BROAD SMILE
↓
Inhale through the nose
↓
Brain
↓
Forehead
↓
Face → Throat → Chest
↓
Upper Abdomen → Lower Abdomen
↓
Pelvic Area
↓
Legs
↓
Arms
↓
BE GRATEFUL

POSITIVE YOGA
PRONE POSTURE

Step-by-Step Instructions:

To begin, lie down on your belly, forehead touching the floor with legs extended and toes pointing outwards. Rest your arms on the sides of your lower body, palms facing upwards and fingers pointing in the direction of the toes. Relax the facial muscles by closing the eyes and releasing the tension in your mind. Bring a smile to your face and concentrate on your spine and shoulder blades.

1. Slowly raise the head, chest and upper body off the floor. Feel the movement in the middle portion of your back and your abdomen.

2. Raise the right arm, rotate and bring it forward in front of you; rest the arm with the palms resting on the floor.

3. Repeat with the left arm.

4. Raise the head, chest and upper body further off the floor, this time supporting yourself on your hands.

5. Now, while concentrating on your shoulder blades, arms and legs; rotate and hold the head as mentioned in steps 6 and 7.

6. Clockwise:

   Rotate head forward with chin touching the collarbone holding to a slow count of ten.

   Rotate the head to the left bringing it closer to the left

shoulder, hold to a slow count of ten.

Move the head further back till it touches the back of the neck, hold up to a slow count of ten.

Rotate head to the right bringing it closer to the right shoulder, hold to a slow count of ten.

7. Anti-Clockwise: Repeat these head rotations in the opposite direction.

Move the head further back till it touches the back of the neck, hold up to a slow count of ten.

Rotate the head to the left bringing it closer to the left shoulder, hold to a slow count of ten.

Rotate head forward with chin touching the collarbone holding to a slow count of ten.

To come back to the original position

8. After the head rotations, raise your head, looking in front of you, slowly come back to the original position by bringing your body down to the floor and arms back to the sides of your body.

9. Bring your arms forward placing and overlapping your hands with palms touching the floor and the back of your hands under your forehead. Turn your head sideways, place it on your overlapping hands.

10. Relax in this position for a minute or so concentrating on the neck and spine.

To finish, come back to a sitting position, take a deep breath, smile and be happy with your accomplishment.

POSITIVE YOGA
SITTING POSTURE

Step-by-Step Instructions:

To begin, sit on the floor with legs extended in front of you and hands resting on the sides of your body, palms touching the floor. Breathe normally. Relax the facial muscles by closing the eyes and releasing the tension in your mind. Bring a smile to your face and concentrate on your spine and shoulder blades.

1. Stretch the neck forward, move head downward so that the chin touches the collar bone. Extend your arms in front of you keeping them straight at the elbows with hands and fingers pointing downwards towards the floor. Feel the stretch at the back of the neck and the upper part of the shoulder blades. Hold up to a slow count of ten; all the time concentrating on your shoulder blades and spinal stretch.

2. Slowly raise your head raising the arms upwards bringing them alongside the ears, keeping them straight at the elbow with palms facing each other. Curl the hands so that the fingers are pointing towards each other. Hold up to a slow count of ten; all the time concentrating on your shoulder blades and spinal stretch.

3. Now bring the arms down sideways parallel to the floor keeping them straight at the elbow with hands and fingers pointing downwards towards the floor. Curl the hands so that the fingers are pointing towards

the body; feel the release of tension as the shoulder blades move towards each other. Hold up to a slow count of ten.

4. Move the arms backwards and further down towards the floor keeping them straight at the elbow with hands and fingers pointing downwards towards the floor. Curl the hands so that the fingers are pointing towards the body. Move the shoulder blades closer and downwards and further experiece the release of energy movement in your entire body. Hold upto a slow count of ten; still concentrating on your shoulder blades and neck stretch.

5. Repeat step 5 by moving the arms further down towards the floor with your fingers almost touching the floor, again holding to a slow count of ten.

   To come back to original sitting position, repeat steps backwards.

6. Repeat step 4

7. Repeat step 3

8. Repeat step 2

9. Repeat step 1

10. Now, for further benefit, repeat steps 1 to 9 at a faster pace, all the time focusing your positive energy towards your neck, shoulder blades and lower spine.

    To finish, come back to the original sitting position, smile and be happy with your accomplishment.

POSITIVE YOGA
STANDING POSTURE

Step-by-Step Instructions:

To begin, stand straight. Breathe normally. Relax the facial muscles by closing your eyes and releasing the tension in your mind. Bring a smile to your face and concentrate on your spine and shoulder blades.

1. Stretch the neck forward, move head downward so that the chin touches the collar bone. Extend your arms in front of you keeping them straight at the elbows with hands and fingers pointing downwards towards the floor. Feel the stretch at the back of the neck and the upper part of the shoulder blades. Hold upto a slow count of ten; concentrate on your shoulder blades and spinal stretch.

2. Slowly raise your head raising the arms upwards bringing them alongside the ears, keeping them straight at the elbow with palms facing each other. Curl the hands so that the fingers are pointing towards each other. Hold up to a slow count of ten.

3. Bring the arms down sideways parallel to the floor keeping them straight at the elbow with hands and fingers pointing downwards towards the floor. Curl the hands so that the fingers are pointing towards the body; feel the release of tension as the shoulder blades move towards each other. Hold upto a slow count of ten.

4. Move the arms backwards and further down towards the floor keeping them straight at the elbow with hands and fingers pointing downwards towards the floor. Curl the hands so that the fingers are pointing towards the body. Move the shoulder blades closer and downwards and further experience the release of energy movement in your entire body. Hold up to a slow count of ten; all the time concentrating on your shoulder blades and neck stretch.

5. Move the arms further down towards the floor, again holding to a slow count of ten.

   To come back to original standing position, repeat steps backwards.

6. Repeat step 4

7. Repeat step 3

8. Repeat step 2

9. Repeat step 1

10. Now, for further benefit, repeat steps 1 to 9 at a faster pace, all the time focusing your positive energy towards your neck, shoulder blades and spine.

    To finish, come back to the original standing position, take a deep breath, smile and be happy with your accomplishment.

POSITIVE YOGA
MEDITATION TECHNIQUE

This technique builds emotional and physical strength by improving focus and concentration. Practicing this meditation technique everyday will vitalize the body internally as well as externally. Concentrating on all body parts, internally cleanses and massages the major organs in our bodies; calming the mind and body by relaxing each part of the body. This meditative technique helps improve overall health.

1. Sit comfortably in a relaxed state of mind. Visualize the flow of positive energy through the internal organs and feel it cleansing each part ,with every breath.
2. Start with focusing on the brain and spinal cord, and relaxing all the nerves throughout your entire body.
3. Then, start relaxing the facial muscles starting with the forehead, going down to the nose, lips, cheeks, chin and jaw line.
4. Next focus on the lungs and heart.
5. Bring back your attention to the mouth, tongue, jaws, going down the esophagus, stomach, pancreas, liver, kidneys, duodenum, intestines and the colon.
6. Focus and relax the genitals and pelvic area.
7. Now, bring your attention upwards and relax the shoulder, upper arms, forearms and hands.
8. Relax the hips, thighs, legs and feet.
9. Let go of all thoughts and emotions; stay calm for about five minutes.
10. Come out of this state by slowly opening your eyes. Smile!

I hope you enjoyed reading this book and sincerely wish that the techniques mentioned will help you achieve your objectives of Health and Wellness.

I wish you a healthy life, filled with positivity and happiness! ☺

NOTES

Chapter 1: Positive Thinking

1. Myers, David G., 2009. Psychology. Ninth Edition, Worth Publishers, Maslow

Chapter 2: Happiness

1. Myers, David G., 2009. Psychology. Ninth Edition, Worth Publishers, *Fight-or-Flight response*

2. Dambrun, M. & Ricard, M., (2011). Self-centeredness and selflessness: A theory of self-based psychological functioning and its consequences for happiness. *Review of General Psychology*, 15(2), 138-157. Retrieved May 6, 2013, from PsycARTICLES database

3. Brazil looks at adding 'happiness' to constitution. Retrieved April 25, 2013, from http://seattletimes.com/html/nationworld/20141028 88_apltbrazillegalizinghappiness.html

4. Uchida, Y. & Kitayama, S. (2009). Happiness and unhappiness in east and west: Themes and variations. *Emotion*, 9(4), 441-456. Retrieved May 6, 2013, from PsycARTICLES database

5. North, R. J., Holahan, C. J., Moos, R. H. & Cronkite, R. C. (2008). Family support, family income, and happiness: A 10-year perspective. *Journal of Family Psychology*, 22(3), 475-483. Retrieved May 6, 2013, from PsycARTICLES database

6. Diener, E., Harter, J., & Arora, R. (2010). Wealth and happiness across the world: Material prosperity predicts life evaluation, whereas psychosocial prosperity predicts positive feeling. *Journal of Personality and Social Psychology,* 99(1), 52-61. Retrieved May 6, 2013, from PsycARTICLES database

7. Cohn, M. A., Fredrickson, B. L., Brown, S. L., Mikels, J. A., & Conway, A. M. (2009). Happiness unpacked: Positive emotions increase life satisfaction by building resilience. *Emotion,* 9(3), 361-368. Retrieved May 6, 2013, from PsycARTICLES database

8. Caprariello, P. A. & Reis, H. T. (2013). To do, to have, or to share? Valuing experiences over material possessions depends on the involvement of others. *Journal of Personality and Social Psychology,* 104(2), 199-215. Retrieved May 6, 2013, from PsycARTICLES database

9. Aknin, L. B., Barrington-Leigh, C. P., Dunn, E.W., Helliwell, J. F., Burns, J., et al. (2013). Prosocial spending and well-being: Cross-cultural evidence for a psychological universal. *Journal of Personality and Social Psychology,* 104(4), 635-652. Retrieved May 6, 2013, from PsycARTICLES database

10. Liberman, V., Boehm, J. K., Lyubomirsky, S. & Ross, L. D. (2009). Happiness and memory: Affective significance of endowment and contrast. *Emotion,* 9(5), 666-680. Retrieved May 6, 2013, from PsycARTICLES database

Chapter 4: Relaxation and Stress Management for Teens and Youth

1. Macan, T. H., Shahani, C., Dipboye, R. L. & Phillips, A. P. (1990). College students' time management: Correlations with academic performance and stress. *Journal of Educational Psychology,* 82(4), 760-768. Retrieved May 14, 2013, from PsycARTICLES database

2. Myers, S. B., Sweeney, A. C., Popick, V., Wesley, K., Bordfeld, A., & Fingerhut, R. (2012). Self-care practices and perceived stress levels among psychology graduate students. *Training and Education in Professional Psychology*, 6(1), 55-66. Retrieved May 14, 2013, from PsycARTICLES database

3. Brand, S., Gerber, M., Pühse, U., & Holsboer-Trachsler, E. (2010). Depression, hypomania, and dysfunctional sleep-related cognitions as mediators between **stress** and insomnia: The best advice is not always found on the pillow! *International Journal of Stress Management*, 17(2), 114-134. Retrieved May 14, 2013, from PsycARTICLES database

SUBJECT INDEX

HAPPINESS